Keto Ninja Foodi Pressure Cooker Cookbook

Easy and Delicious Ketogenic Recipes for a Healthy Lifestyle (Burn Fat, Balance Hormones and Reverse Disease)

Pamelen Glonk

Table of Contents

Introduction

A balanced diet coupled with regular exercise is the best way to keep our body healthy.

All of us need to eat every day, which is why we should be mindful of what we consume.

Some people who have existing medical conditions or food allergies often require a special diet to help manage their disease.

Others take on a diet for reasons like weight management, reducing the risk of chronic illnesses, improving vitality, and treating digestive problems.

Food choices are also greatly influenced by one's culture, religion, lifestyle, and ethical practices.

There are so many diet plans you can choose from to match your goals. One popular diet plan that has been recently making waves in the last few years is the ketogenic diet.

Chapter 1: Understanding the Keto Diet

The History of Keto

The low-carb high-fat diet was first used in the 1920s as an effective treatment for epilepsy, particularly in drug-resistance.

Most patients reported lesser seizures and improved alertness. The keto diet is intended to induce ketosis by consuming less carbohydrate and more fat. Dr. Russell Wilder devised the classic ketogenic diet that follows a 4:1 ratio between fat and carbs/protein.

In a classic keto diet, fat would account for 90 percent, protein for 6 percent, and carbohydrates the remaining 4 percent.

The Process of Ketosis

It is the sugar in the food we eat that provides our body with the energy to function as it should. The hormone insulin helps the cells absorb glucose (sugar) to use as fuel. It also signals the body to store excess glucose in the liver as glycogen and muscles as fat to use in the future.

When the body is not getting enough glucose, it can tap into a backup energy source - fat. This is a metabolic state known as ketosis.

Ketosis produces an acid called ketone that builds up in the bloodstream and is expelled through urine.

Ketones can give a more efficient fuel source for the body, and most especially the brain.

Reaching Ketosis

Aside from minimizing our intake of carbs, we can also reach ketosis when we increase our consumption of healthy fats, moderate amounts of protein, exercising, and fasting. Adopting a ketogenic diet is one way to keep the body in ketosis.

It is important to mention that the presence of too much ketone in the body can be dangerous and may result in a condition called ketoacidosis. One way to avoid this is by consulting with a dietician or health professional before trying the keto diet.

Benefits of Ketogenic Diet

Most people prefer the keto diet for weight loss as it makes their body utilize and burn the fat without them feeling hungry, as is the case with other diets.

People on a keto diet reported feeling fuller, an aspect that may help with obesity and food addiction. Weight loss also immediately improves blood pressure levels for people suffering from high blood pressure.

Insulin is the body's fat-storing hormone. By decreasing your carbohydrate intake, you will also decrease the levels of insulin that will let you access your body's stored fats. Increasing your consumption of good fats will reduce the risk of strokes and heart problems.

The keto diet also helps keep blood sugar stable in diabetic patients and prevent prediabetes. Apart from weight loss, the ketogenic diet has other health benefits, especially in managing epilepsy.

There are recent studies of the keto diet as therapy for a range of neurological conditions such as autism, brain injury, brain tumors, gliomas, stroke, multiple sclerosis, migraine, ALS, Parkinson's, and Alzheimer's that are showing great promise.

Chapter 2: Ninja Foodi Pressure Cooker Basics

What is the Ninja Foodi?

The Ninja Foodi is a tabletop multi-cooker that can complete up to nine functions such as pressure cook, sear/sauté, air crisp, slow cook, broil, bake, steam, dehydrate, and yogurt.

What is TenderCrisp Technology?

Ninja Foodi's proprietary TenderCrisp Technology is a 2-step cooking process that involves pressure cooking and air crisping.

By initially cooking with pressure, you get food that is tender and juicy. The pressure also helps the flavors and aromas get absorbed within the food.

Then by switching to the air crisp function, the dry and hot air will fully circulate to give you even browning and scrumptious flavors known as the Maillard reaction.

Benefits of Ninja Foodi

Apart from getting nine different cooking functions in a single appliance, the Ninja Foodi is perfect if you're planning to try the keto diet.

The Ninja Foodi will make cooking effortless as it can handle frozen food, cook it until its tender, then give it that delectable crisp at the end. You'll be able to enjoy flavorful meals quicker and with much less effort than if you would cook these with a stove or oven.

The Ninja Foodi has great reviews online. Users are raving about the TenderCrisp technology since the Foodi is the only pressure cooker that can also air fry.

It even has an active online community where you can ask for tips, share and get amazing recipes, and gain access to exclusive offers and giveaways.

The Ninja Foodi comes with UL-certified safety mechanisms, a 1-year VIP elite service warranty, and a 90-day money back guarantee. It also includes a cookbook with up to 50 wonderful recipes you will surely love.

Chapter 3: Food to Eat and Food to Avoid

The ketogenic diet follows a few basic principles: consuming a high amount of fat and non-starchy vegetables, a moderate quantity of proteins, and a very low amount of carbohydrates. Below are foods you can eat on a keto diet.

1. Seafood and fatty fish

These types of food are the top choices for the keto diet since they are filled with good fat and are free from carbohydrates. Aim to consume at least two servings of fish per week like salmon, mackerel, sardines, cod, flounder, catfish, halibut, snapper, tuna, and mahi-mahi. It is important to note that some shellfishes have carbohydrates like mussels and clams.

2. Fats and oils

Butter, coconut oil, MCT oil, ghee, lard, olive oil, avocado oil, and macadamia nut oil are great options. Extra virgin olive oil is rich in oleic acid and phenols that promote heart health. Coconut oil contains MCT or medium-chain triglycerides that are converted into ketones by the liver.

3. Low-carb vegetables

An easy trick to remember is to only eat vegetables that grow above the ground and those that are dark-green and leafy. Root crops, like potatoes, are full of carbohydrates and should be avoided. Choose non-starchy vegetables that are also high in essential nutrients like cabbage, cauliflower, broccoli, green beans, Swiss chard, kale, and spinach.

4. Meat and poultry

Moderate amounts of protein is a key part of the keto diet. Unprocessed meat should be eaten instead of processed or cured since it has added sugars. Choose fatty portions of beef and pork. Bacon is one of the favorite options of keto dieters under this category. You may also eat offal and organs such as liver and heart as they are good sources of proteins and vitamins. Aside from chicken, you may also choose darker meats like duck, turkey, quail, and pheasant.

5. Eggs

Whole eggs are also wonderful sources of protein and fat. Whenever possible, opt for free-range and organic. Cook them however you like, as they also promote eye and heart health.

6. Cheese and dairy

One of the best things about the keto diet is that it allows you to eat foods that are often avoided in other diets like fat and cheese. Cheeses are good sources of fatty acids, proteins, vitamins A and B, and calcium. Choose high-fat hard cheeses like aged cheddar, feta, Swiss, gouda, and parmesan since they contain less carbs. Similarly, opt for full-fat versions of yogurt and cream.

7. Avocados and berries

You will not see much of fruits in the ketogenic diet as they are loaded with sugars. However, avocados and berries are great choices since they are low in carbohydrates and are filled with nutrients. Avocados help lower bad cholesterol and increase the amount of good cholesterol. Berries such as blackberries, blueberries, strawberries, and raspberries, are rich in antioxidants that fight off inflammations and diseases. Coconut meat and lemon are also terrific choices.

8. Dark chocolate

Cocoa is rich in antioxidants that help reduce the risk of heart diseases and improve blood circulation. Choose dark chocolate that contains at least 70 percent cocoa.

9. Unsweetened beverages

Just because you can't have sugar doesn't mean that you'll have to ditch your favourite beverages. You can still drink coffee and tea as long as you stay away from sugar, sweeteners, and milk. Butter coffee is popular among keto dieters since it helps improve mental clarity and cognitive functions. Caffeine not only gives you the needed boost, but it has also shown to reduce the risk of diabetes, stroke, and some forms of cancer.

Since we are aiming to power our body with fat instead of sugar, the foods you should avoid are those with carbohydrates. Avoid these foods when in a keto diet.

1. Starchy vegetables

Potatoes, sweet potatoes, corn, yams, and taro have high amounts of carbohydrates.

2. Fresh fruits

Fruits like apples, pears, pineapples, bananas, and mangos have high levels of sugar.

3. Grains

Rice, pasta, bread, wheat, flour, oats, rye, oatmeal, buckwheat, quinoa, chips, crackers, cereals, and barley are some examples of foods to avoid under this category.

4. Sweetened beverages and all kinds of sweeteners

Avoid fruit juices, hot chocolate, sodas, beer, and cocktails. Sugars, honey, maple syrup, and other sweeteners should also be avoided completely.

Chapter 4: 30-Day Meal Plan

Week 1

Sunday

Breakfast: Breakfast bacon & green beans

Lunch: Rosemary chicken

Dinner: Salmon & asparagus

Monday

Breakfast: Creamy frittata

Lunch: Spaghetti marinara

Dinner: Chicken with garlic butter

Tuesday

Breakfast: Breakfast cauliflower casserole

Lunch: Crab legs

Dinner: Lamb stew

Wednesday

Breakfast: Soft boiled eggs

Lunch: Savory turkey breast

Dinner: Cheesy green beans

Thursday

Breakfast: Shakshuka with kale

Lunch: Fish Curry

Dinner: Mexican beef

Friday

Breakfast: Spinach frittata

Lunch: Chicken barbeque

Dinner: Beef short ribs

Saturday

Breakfast: Breakfast sausage casserole

Lunch: Lamb shanks

Dinner: Shredded chicken

Week 2

Sunday

Breakfast: Shakshuka with kale

Lunch: Pork taco bowl

Dinner: Crab legs

Monday

Breakfast: Egg bites

Lunch: Southern cabbage

Dinner: Pot roast with gravy

Tuesday

Breakfast: Keto quiche

Lunch: Spicy fish stew

Dinner: Pork belly

Wednesday

Breakfast: Egg & veggie cups

Lunch: Lamb curry

Dinner: Chili lime steak

Thursday

Breakfast: Breakfast cauliflower casserole

Lunch: Beef stroganoff

Dinner: Shrimp & broccoli

Friday

Breakfast: Sausage & spinach casserole

Lunch: Beef short ribs

Dinner: Fish with black bean & ginger

Saturday

Breakfast: Breakfast burrito in a bowl

Lunch: Brussels sprouts

Dinner: Coconut lemon turkey

Week 3

Sunday

Breakfast: Shakshuka with kale

Lunch: Braised beef

Dinner: Cauliflower soup

Monday

Breakfast: Breakfast bacon & green beans

Lunch: Savory collard greens

Dinner: Jamaican jerk pork roast

Tuesday

Breakfast: Egg bites

Lunch: Chicken adobo

Dinner: Beef stroganoff

Wednesday

Breakfast: Keto quiche

Lunch: Butter chicken

Dinner: Pork stew

Thursday

Breakfast: Egg & veggie cups

Lunch: Chicken tikka masala

Dinner: Rosemary lamb

Friday

Breakfast: Creamy frittata

Lunch: Lamb curry

Dinner: Mashed cauliflower potatoes

Saturday

Breakfast: Breakfast sausage casserole

Lunch: Butternut squash soup

Dinner: Pot roast with gravy

Week 4

Sunday

Breakfast: Breakfast cauliflower casserole

Lunch: Fish saag

Dinner: Vietnamese pork tenderloin

Monday

Breakfast: Keto quiche

Lunch: Coconut lemon turkey

Dinner: Shrimp & broccoli

Tuesday

Breakfast: Soft boiled eggs

Lunch: Chicken tikka masala

Dinner: Pork carnitas

Wednesday

Breakfast: Spinach frittata

Lunch: Creamy shrimp

Dinner: Lamb shanks

Thursday

Breakfast: Sausage & spinach casserole

Lunch: Turkey buffalo meatballs

Dinner: Kale & cauliflower soup

Friday

Breakfast: Egg bites

Lunch: Spaghetti marinara

Dinner: Lemon herbed salmon

Saturday

Breakfast: Sausage & spinach casserole

Lunch: Chicken adobo

Dinner: Fish saag

Chapter 5: Breakfast

Soft Boiled Eggs

Preparation Time: 2 minutes
Cooking Time: 3 minutes
Servings: 4

Ingredients:

- 2 cups water
- 4 eggs
- 1 bowl cold water

Method:

1. Add water to the Ninja Foodi.
2. Place the steamer insert inside the pot.
3. Add the eggs to the steamer.
4. Seal the pot.
5. Cook on low for 3 minutes.
6. Release pressure naturally.
7. Transfer the eggs to the bowl with cold water.

Serving Suggestions: Serve with toasted bread.

Preparation & Cooking Tips: Let the eggs cool for 10 minutes before serving.

Spinach Frittata

Preparation Time: 10 minutes
Cooking Time: 5 minutes
Servings: 4

Ingredients:

- Cooking spray
- 6 eggs, beaten
- 1 teaspoon onion, minced
- ¼ cup tomato, diced
- ½ cup spinach, chopped
- ½ teaspoon garlic powder
- Salt and pepper to taste
- 1 cup water

Method:

1. Spray the pot with oil.
2. Combine the rest of the ingredients except water in a ramekin.
3. Place the steamer inside the Ninja Foodi.
4. Add the ramekin to the steamer.
5. Pour the water into the pot.
6. Seal the pot.
7. Cook on low for 5 minutes.
8. Release pressure naturally.

Serving Suggestions: Serve with toasted bread and salad.

Preparation & Cooking Tips: You can also use garlic salt in lieu of garlic powder and salt.

Breakfast Bacon & Green Beans

Preparation Time: 10 minutes
Cooking Time: 10 minutes
Servings: 6

Ingredients:

- 1 cup onion, chopped
- 6 cups green beans, sliced in half
- 5 slices bacon
- Salt and pepper to taste
- ¼ cup water

Method:

1. Set the Ninja Foodi to sauté.
2. Cook the bacon in the pot until crispy.
3. Transfer to a cutting board and let cool.
4. Once cool, chop into smaller pieces.
5. Add the onion and green beans to the pot.
6. Cook for 2 minutes, stirring.
7. Season with salt and pepper.
8. Pour in the water.
9. Seal the pot.
10. Cook on high for 2 minutes.
11. Release pressure quickly.
12. Stir in the bacon before serving.

Serving Suggestions: Sprinkle with Parmesan cheese before serving.

Preparation & Cooking Tips: You can also skip the sauté and pressure cook the ingredients directly.

Breakfast Sausage Casserole

Preparation Time: 10 minutes
Cooking Time: 30 minutes
Servings: 6

Ingredients:

- 1 lb. ground Italian sausage
- 4 eggs
- 2/3 cup cheddar cheese, grated
- 2/3 cup low-sodium chicken broth
- 1 cup water

Method:

1. Set your Ninja Foodi to sauté.
2. Cook the sausage until browned.
3. Combine the sausage and remaining ingredients except water in a small baking pan.
4. Add a steamer inside the pot.
5. Place the baking pan on top of the steamer.
6. Pour the water into the bottom of the pot.
7. Seal the pot.
8. Cook on high for 5 minutes.
9. Release pressure naturally.

Serving Suggestions: Garnish with chopped green onion.

Preparation & Cooking Tips: You can also use turkey sausage for this recipe.

Breakfast Cauliflower Casserole

Preparation Time: 10 minutes
Cooking Time: 20 minutes
Servings: 6

Ingredients:

- 6 eggs, beaten
- ½ cup milk
- ½ teaspoon ground paprika
- ½ teaspoon dried oregano
- Salt to taste
- Cooking spray
- 1 cup cauliflower florets
- 1 red bell pepper, chopped
- 2 green onions, chopped
- ¼ cup bacon, cooked and chopped
- 1 cup cheddar cheese, grated
- 1 cup water

Method:

1. In a bowl, mix the eggs and milk.
2. Season with the paprika, oregano and salt.
3. Mix well.
4. Spray small cake pan with oil.
5. Arrange the remaining ingredients except water in layers.
6. Add the egg mixture on top.
7. Cover with foil.
8. Pour water into the pot.
9. Place cake pan on a steamer inside the Ninja Foodi.
10. Cook on high for 20 minutes.

Serving Suggestions: Sprinkle with Parmesan cheese before serving.

Preparation & Cooking Tips: You can also use cooked turkey bacon for this recipe.

Creamy Frittata

Preparation Time: 15 minutes
Cooking Time: 12 minutes
Servings: 8

Ingredients:

- 8 eggs, beaten
- 1 onion, minced
- 1 bell pepper, diced
- ¼ cup cream
- ¼ cup cheddar cheese, shredded
- Salt and pepper to taste
- 1 cup water

Method:

1. Mix all the ingredients except water in a bowl.
2. Transfer to a small baking pan.
3. Pour water into the Ninja Foodi.
4. Place a steamer inside.
5. Add the baking pan to the steamer.
6. Seal the pot.
7. Cook on high for 12 minutes.
8. Release pressure naturally.

Serving Suggestions: Serve with sour cream.

Preparation & Cooking Tips: You can add a pinch of chili powder to the frittata if you like.

Egg Bites

Preparation Time: 10 minutes
Cooking Time: 15 minutes
Servings: 14

Ingredients:

- Cooking spray
- 10 eggs, beaten
- ½ cup cheddar cheese, grated
- 8 slices bacon, cooked crisp and crumbled
- ½ cup cream
- 1 teaspoon dried basil
- Salt and pepper to taste
- 1 cup water

Method:

1. Spray small muffin pan with cooking spray.
2. Combine all the ingredients except water in a bowl.
3. Pour mixture into the muffin cups.
4. Cover with foil.
5. Add water to the pot.
6. Add steamer inside the pot.
7. Place the muffin pan on top of the steamer.
8. Seal the pot.
9. Cook on high for 14 minutes.
10. Release pressure quickly.

Serving Suggestions: Garnish with chopped chives.

Preparation & Cooking Tips: You can also use coconut milk instead of cream.

Egg & Veggie Cups

Preparation Time: 5 minutes
Cooking Time: 10 minutes
Servings: 4

Ingredients:

- 4 eggs, beaten
- 1 onion, chopped
- 1 tomato, chopped
- ½ cup mushrooms
- 1 bell pepper, chopped
- ¼ cup half and half
- ½ cup cheddar cheese, shredded
- Salt and pepper to taste
- 2 tablespoons cilantro, chopped
- 2 cups water

Method:

1. Mix all the ingredients except water in a large bowl.
2. Transfer mixture to glass jars with lids.
3. Seal the jars.
4. Add water to the Ninja Foodi.
5. Place a steamer inside.
6. Add the jars on top of the steamer.
7. Cook on high for 5 minutes.
8. Release pressure quickly.

Serving Suggestions: Top with cheese before serving.

Preparation & Cooking Tips: You can also add chopped carrots to the mixture.

Shakshuka with Kale

Preparation Time: 10 minutes
Cooking Time: 15 minutes
Servings: 4

Ingredients:

- 1 tablespoon olive oil
- ½ onion, diced
- 2 cloves garlic, minced
- ½ red bell pepper, diced
- ½ teaspoon paprika
- 1 teaspoon chili powder
- ½ teaspoon ground cumin
- Salt and pepper to taste
- 2 cups kale, chopped
- 1 ½ cups marinara sauce
- 4 eggs

Method:

1. Set your Ninja Foodi to sauté.
2. Pour the oil and cook the onion, garlic and bell pepper for 3 minutes.
3. Season with the spices, salt and pepper.
4. Cook for 3 minutes.
5. Stir in the kale and cook for 1 minute.
6. Add the marinara sauce and stir.
7. Crack the eggs on top.
8. Lock the lid in place.
9. Cook on high for 1 minute.

Serving Suggestions: Garnish with chopped parsley.

Preparation & Cooking Tips: Serve with toasted French bread slices.

Sausage & Spinach Casserole

Preparation Time: 10 minutes
Cooking Time: 2 hours
Servings: 4

Ingredients:

- 1 teaspoon oil
- 8 oz. sausage links
- 8 eggs, beaten
- ½ onion, chopped
- 1 bell pepper, chopped
- 1 tomato, diced
- 2 oz. cheese
- ½ cup spinach, chopped
- ¼ cup milk
- Salt and pepper to taste
- 1 ½ cup water

Method:

1. Add oil to the Ninja Foodi.
2. Set it to sauté.
3. Cook the sausage until browned. Drain the fat.
4. Mix the remaining ingredients except water in a bowl.
5. Add to the Ninja Foodi along with the sausage.
6. Slow cook for 2 hours.

Serving Suggestions: Garnish with onion rings.

Preparation & Cooking Tips: You can also pressure cook the casserole on high setting for 10 minutes, but place mixture in a baking pan on top of a steamer, with 1 cup water inside the pot.

Breakfast Burrito in a Bowl

Preparation Time: 10 minutes
Cooking Time: 15 minutes
Servings: 4

Ingredients:

- 6 eggs
- 3 tablespoons butter
- Salt and pepper to taste
- ½ lb. breakfast sausage, cooked
- ½ cup cheddar cheese, shredded
- 1 avocado, sliced into cubes
- ½ cup sour cream
- ½ cup salsa

Method:

1. Beat the eggs in a bowl.
2. Stir in the butter and season with salt and pepper.
3. Set Ninja Foodi to sauté.
4. Pour in the egg mixture to the pot.
5. Cook for 5 minutes.
6. Stir in the cheese and sausage.
7. Transfer mixture to bowls.
8. Top each bowl with the remaining ingredients.

Serving Suggestions: Top with chopped green onion before serving.

Preparation & Cooking Tips: You can also use Italian sausage or turkey sausage for this recipe.

Keto Quiche

Preparation Time: 10 minutes
Cooking Time: 30 minutes
Servings: 6

Ingredients:

- Cooking spray
- 1 ½ cups water
- 6 eggs, beaten
- ½ cup spinach, chopped
- ¾ cup heavy cream
- ½ cup feta cheese, crumbled
- ¾ cup gouda, shredded
- ¼ cup sun dried tomatoes, chopped
- 1 teaspoon rosemary, chopped
- Salt and pepper to taste

Method:

1. Spray a soufflé dish with oil.
2. Place this inside the Ninja Foodi on top of the steamer.
3. Add water to the pot.
4. Combine the remaining ingredients in a bowl.
5. Transfer to the soufflé dish.
6. Seal the pot.
7. Cook on high for 30 minutes.
8. Release pressure quickly.

Serving Suggestions: Garnish with chopped parsley.

Preparation & Cooking Tips: You can also add a pinch of red pepper flakes to the mixture.

Chapter 6: Snack & Appetizer

Paneer Indian Soft Cheese

Preparation Time: 2 hours and 10 minutes
Cooking Time: 10 minutes
Servings: 6 ounces

Ingredients:

- ¼ cup white vinegar
- 1 quart half and half

Method:

1. Add vinegar and half and half to the Ninja Foodi.
2. Seal the pot.
3. Cook on low for 4 minutes.
4. Release pressure naturally.
5. Strain mixture through a cheese cloth.
6. Let the cheese curds form for 1 to 2 hours.

Serving Suggestions: Serve cheese with crackers.

Stuffed Tomatoes

Preparation Time: 20 minutes
Cooking Time: 15 minutes
Servings: 4

Ingredients:

- 4 tomatoes, tops sliced off and pulp removed
- Salt and pepper to taste
- 10 oz. spinach, chopped
- 5 oz. garlic and herb cheese
- 3 tablespoons sour cream
- ½ cup Parmesan cheese, grated

Method:

1. Season the tomatoes with salt and pepper.
2. Mix the remaining ingredients in a bowl.
3. Stuff the tomatoes with this mixture.
4. Add the air fryer basket to the Ninja Foodi.
5. Seal the pot.
6. Air fry at 350 degrees F for 15 minutes.

Serving Suggestions: Sprinkle with dried herbs on top of before serving.

Preparation & Cooking Tips: You can also top the stuffed tomatoes with mozzarella cheese.

Spiced Eggplant

Preparation Time: 20 minutes
Cooking Time: 5 minutes
Servings: 6

Ingredients:

- ¼ cup vegetable oil, divided
- 1 eggplant, sliced
- ½ onion, diced
- 3 cloves garlic, minced
- Pinch cayenne pepper
- ¼ teaspoon turmeric
- ¼ cup tomatoes, chopped
- Salt to taste
- ¼ teaspoon liquid smoke
- ½ cup water

Method:

1. Set the Ninja Foodi to sauté.
2. Pour 2 tablespoons oil to the pot.
3. Cook the eggplant for 15 minutes.
4. Stir in the remaining ingredients.
5. Close the pot.
6. Cook on high for 3 minutes.

Serving Suggestions: Garnish with cilantro.

Preparation & Cooking Tips: Skip cayenne pepper if you don't want the eggplant to be too spicy.

Beet Dip

Preparation Time: 5 minutes
Cooking Time: 10 minutes
Servings: 4

Ingredients:

- 1 ½ cups water
- 2 beets, sliced
- 1 cup Greek yogurt
- 2 cloves garlic, minced
- Salt to taste
- 2 tablespoons lemon juice
- ¼ cup dill, chopped

Method:

1. Pour the water into the Ninja Foodi.
2. Add the steamer inside.
3. Place the beets on top of the steamer.
4. Seal and cook on high for 10 minutes.
5. Release pressure naturally.
6. Let cool.
7. Add beets to a food processor.
8. Process until smooth.
9. Stir in the remaining ingredients.

Serving Suggestions: Sprinkle with white sesame seeds before serving.

Preparation & Cooking Tips: You can also use labneh in place of yogurt.

Garlic Spaghetti Squash

Preparation Time: 2 minutes
Cooking Time: 17 minutes
Servings: 4

Ingredients:

- ½ spaghetti squash
- 1 ½ cups water
- 3 tablespoons olive oil
- 8 cloves garlic, minced
- 4 cups fresh spinach, chopped
- Salt to taste
- ½ cup almonds, slivered

Method:

1. Pierce the squash with a fork or knife.
2. Add water to the Ninja Foodi.
3. Place the steamer inside.
4. Add the squash on top of the steamer.
5. Seal the pot.
6. Cook on high for 7 minutes. Let cool.
7. Scrape the squash to create strands. Set aside.
8. Set the Ninja Foodi to sauté.
9. Add the oil and cook the garlic and spinach for 2 minutes.
10. Stir in the spaghetti squash.
11. Season with salt.
12. Top with almonds.

Serving Suggestions: Sprinkle with Parmesan cheese.

Preparation & Cooking Tips: You can also use chopped walnuts in place of almonds.

Cauliflower Mac & Cheese

Preparation Time: 5 minutes
Cooking Time: 15 minutes
Servings: 2

Ingredients:

- 2 cups cauliflower rice
- 2 tablespoons cream cheese
- ½ cup half and half
- ½ cup cheddar cheese, shredded
- Salt and pepper to taste
- 1 ½ cups water

Method:

1. Combine all the ingredients in a heatproof bowl.
2. Cover bowl with foil.
3. Add the water to the Ninja Foodi.
4. Place the steamer inside the pot.
5. Add the bowl on top of the steamer.
6. Seal the pot.
7. Cook on high for 5 minutes.
8. Release pressure naturally.

Serving Suggestions: Garnish with chopped herbs.

Preparation & Cooking Tips: You can also sprinkle cheddar cheese on top once done, and broil in the oven for 5 minutes.

Zucchini Lasagna

Preparation Time: 15 minutes
Cooking Time: 20 minutes
Servings: 4

Ingredients:

- 2 cups water
- Cooking spray
- 1 cup marinara sauce
- 1 zucchini, sliced into thin strips

Meat

- 1 cup onions, chopped
- 2 cloves garlic, minced
- ½ lb. Italian sausage

Cheese

- ½ cup Parmesan cheese, shredded
- ½ cup mozzarella cheese, shredded
- ½ cup ricotta cheese
- 1 eggs, beaten
- ½ teaspoon Italian seasoning
- ½ teaspoon garlic, minced
- Pepper to taste

Method:

1. Spray small baking pan with oil.
2. Arrange zucchini slices in a small baking pan.
3. Spread a layer of marinara sauce on top.
4. Sprinkle onion, garlic and sausage on top of sauce.
5. Repeat layers.
6. In another bowl, mix the cheese ingredients.
7. Add this on top of the sausage.
8. Cover the pan with foil.

9. Add water to the Ninja Foodi.
10. Place the steamer inside.
11. Add the pan on top of the steamer.
12. Seal the pot.
13. Cook on high for 20 minutes.
14. Release pressure naturally.

Serving Suggestions: Garnish with chopped fresh herbs.

Preparation & Cooking Tips: Be sure to use low-sugar marinara sauce.

Creamy Eggplant Appetizer

Preparation Time: 5 minutes
Cooking Time: 20 minutes
Servings: 6

Ingredients:

- 3 cups eggplant, chopped
- ½ teaspoon oil
- ½ teaspoon garam masala
- ¼ teaspoon turmeric
- Salt to taste
- 1 tablespoon oil
- 1 onion, sliced
- ¼ cup water
- ¼ cup cream

Method:

1. Toss eggplant in oil.
2. Season with garam masala, turmeric and salt.
3. Set Ninja Foodi to sauté.
4. Cook onion for 2 minutes.
5. Stir in eggplant.
6. Cook for 10 minutes.
7. Pour in water.
8. Cook for 3 minutes.
9. Stir in cream before serving.

Serving Suggestions: Sprinkle with chopped green onion.

Preparation & Cooking Tips: You can also add more spices if you want your appetizer tastier.

Spinach Artichoke Dip

Preparation Time: 10 minutes
Cooking Time: 20 minutes
Servings: 10

Ingredients:

- ½ cup chicken broth
- 3 oz. canned green chili
- 13 oz. canned artichoke hearts, drained and chopped
- 8 oz. cream cheese
- ½ cup mayonnaise
- ½ cup sour cream
- 10 oz. spinach, chopped
- ½ teaspoon garlic
- ½ teaspoon onion powder
- Salt to taste
- 3 cups mozzarella cheese, grated
- 1 ½ cups Parmesan cheese, grated

Method:

1. Add all the ingredients except the cheeses to the Ninja Foodi.
2. Mix well.
3. Seal the pot.
4. Cook on high for 4 minutes.
5. Release pressure quickly.
6. Stir in the cheeses.

Serving Suggestions: Serve with keto chips.

Preparation & Cooking Tips: You can also add a pinch of cayenne pepper if you like your dip spicy.

Chicken Enchilada Dip

Preparation Time: 5 minutes
Cooking Time: 15 minutes
Servings: 12

Ingredients:

- 2 chicken breasts
- 1 ½ cups enchilada sauce
- 8 oz. cream cheese
- 1 ½ cups Mexican cheese blend
- Hot sauce

Method:

1. Add the chicken to the Ninja Foodi.
2. Pour the sauce on top.
3. Seal the pot.
4. Cook on high for 12 minutes.
5. Release pressure quickly.
6. Shred chicken.
7. Put it back to the pot.
8. Stir in the rest of the ingredients.
9. Seal the pot.
10. Cook on high for 2 minutes.

Serving Suggestions: Serve with keto chips or vegetable dippers.

Preparation & Cooking Tips: You can double or triple the recipe if you're having a big party.

Meatball Appetizers

Preparation Time: 15 minutes
Cooking Time: 15 minutes
Servings: 6

Ingredients:

- 1 ¼ lb. ground pork
- 2 strips bacon, chopped
- 1 egg, beaten
- ½ onion, minced
- 2 tablespoons almond flour
- 1 clove garlic, minced
- Salt and pepper to taste
- 2 tablespoons avocado oil
- 1 cup chicken broth

Method:

1. Combine all the ingredients except oil and stock.
2. Form meatballs from the mixture.
3. Set the Ninja Foodi to sauté.
4. Pour oil into the pot.
5. Cook the meatballs until browned.
6. Pour broth into the pot.
7. Seal the pot.
8. Cook on high for 7 minutes.

Serving Suggestions: Serve with pepper sauce.

Preparation & Cooking Tips: Insert toothpicks into the meatballs.

Cheesy Meatballs

Preparation Time: 15 minutes
Cooking Time: 5 minutes
Servings: 16

Ingredients:

- 1 lb. ground beef
- ½ cup almond flour
- ¼ cup Parmesan cheese, shredded
- 1 tablespoon Italian Seasoning
- 1 clove garlic, minced
- Salt and pepper to taste
- 3 oz. cheese, sliced into cubes
- 4 cups marinara sauce

Method:

1. Combine all ingredients except cheese and marinara sauce in a bowl.
2. Refrigerate the mixture for 10 minutes.
3. Form meatballs from the mixture.
4. Insert cheese cubes into the meatballs.
5. Pour the marina sauce into the Ninja Foodi.
6. Place the meatballs on top of the sauce.
7. Seal the pot.
8. Cook on high for 8 minutes.

Serving Suggestions: Garnish with chopped parsley.

Preparation & Cooking Tips: Use low-carb marinara sauce.

Chapter 7: Vegetarian

Southern Cabbage

Preparation Time: 20 minutes
Cooking Time: 15 minutes
Servings: 8

Ingredients:

- 3 slices bacon
- 1 head cabbage, cored and sliced
- ¼ cup butter
- 2 cups chicken broth
- Salt and pepper to taste

Method:

1. Set Ninja Foodi to sauté.
2. Add the bacon and cook for 5 minutes.
3. Stir in the butter and cabbage.
4. Add the chicken broth.
5. Season with salt and pepper.
6. Seal the pot.
7. Cook on low for 3 minutes.
8. Release pressure quickly.

Serving Suggestions: Sprinkle with pepper before serving.

Preparation & Cooking Tips: Use low-sodium chicken broth.

Brussels Sprouts

Preparation Time: 10 minutes
Cooking Time: 3 minutes
Servings: 4

Ingredients:

- 2 tablespoons coconut oil
- ½ cup onion, chopped
- 2 teaspoons garlic, minced
- 3 strips bacon, sliced
- 1 lb. Brussels sprouts
- ½ cup water
- Salt and pepper to taste

Method:

1. Set your Ninja Foodi to sauté.
2. Pour the coconut oil into the pot.
3. Cook the onion, garlic and bacon for 3 minutes.
4. Stir in the Brussels sprouts and water.
5. Season with the salt and pepper.
6. Close the pot.
7. Cook on low for 3 minutes.
8. Release pressure quickly.

Serving Suggestions: Drizzle with melted butter before serving.

Preparation & Cooking Tips: You can also add Parmesan cheese into the mix.

Mashed Cauliflower Potatoes

Preparation Time: 5 minutes
Cooking Time: 5 minutes
Servings: 4

Ingredients:

- 1 cup water
- 4 cups cauliflower florets
- 1 tablespoon butter
- ¼ teaspoon garlic powder
- 1 tablespoon chives, chopped
- Salt and pepper to taste

Method:

1. Place the steamer inside the Ninja Foodi.
2. Pour in the water to the bottom of the pot.
3. Add the cauliflower to the steamer.
4. Seal the pot.
5. Cook on high for 5 minutes.
6. Release pressure quickly.
7. Mash the cauliflower.
8. Stir in the butter
9. Add butter, garlic powder, chives, salt and pepper.

Serving Suggestions: Sprinkle with chopped parsley before serving.

Preparation & Cooking Tips: You can also season the cauliflower with pepper.

Spaghetti Marinara

Preparation Time: 5 minutes
Cooking Time: 10 minutes
Servings: 4

Ingredients:

- 1 teaspoon olive oil
- 1 onion, chopped
- 4 cups cooked spaghetti squash
- 1 cup low-carb marinara sauce
- 1 teaspoon dried oregano
- Salt and pepper to taste

Method:

1. Set the Ninja Foodi to sauté.
2. Add the olive oil to the pot.
3. Cook the onion for 1 minute, stirring often.
4. Add the remaining ingredients.
5. Cook for 2 minutes.

Serving Suggestions: Top with black olives and sprinkle with Parmesan cheese.

Preparation & Cooking Tips: Use the previous spaghetti squash recipe to prepare the noodles for this recipe.

Cheesy Green Beans

Preparation Time: 10 minutes
Cooking Time: 15 minutes
Servings: 6

Ingredients:

- 1 tablespoon olive oil
- 1 cup onion, chopped
- 6 cups green beans, sliced in half
- Salt and pepper to taste
- ¼ cup water
- 1 tablespoon Parmesan cheese
- ½ cup mozzarella cheese

Method:

1. Set your Ninja Foodi to sauté.
2. Add the oil and onion.
3. Cook while stirring for 1 minute.
4. Add the green beans, and cook while stirring for another 1 minute.
5. Season with salt and pepper.
6. Pour in the water.
7. Seal the pot.
8. Cook on high for 4 minutes.
9. Release pressure quickly.
10. Sprinkle with Parmesan cheese and mozzarella cheese.
11. Let mozzarella cheese melt before serving.

Serving Suggestions: Sprinkle with dried herbs before serving.

Preparation & Cooking Tips: You can also cook green beans in advance and reheat with the cheese when ready to serve.

Cauliflower Soup

Preparation Time: 15 minutes
Cooking Time: 20 minutes
Servings: 6

Ingredients:

- 1 tablespoon olive oil
- ¼ cup onion, chopped
- 3 cloves garlic, minced
- 1 stalk celery, chopped
- Salt and pepper to taste
- 3 cups chicken broth
- 6 cups cauliflower florets
- ¾ cup sour cream
- 1 ½ cups Monterey Jack cheese, shredded

Method:

1. Add oil to the Ninja Foodi.
2. Set it to sauté.
3. Cook onion, garlic and celery for 4 minutes.
4. Season with salt and pepper.
5. Pour in the broth.
6. Add the cauliflower.
7. Seal the pot.
8. Cook on high for 5 minutes.
9. Release pressure naturally.
10. Let cool.
11. Transfer contents of pot to a food processor.
12. Pulse until smooth.
13. Put mixture back to the pot.
14. Add remaining ingredients.
15. Season with salt and pepper.
16. Heat for 5 minutes before serving.

Serving Suggestions: Sprinkle with green onions.

Preparation & Cooking Tips: You can make this soup ahead, freezer and reheat for later use.

Savory Collard Greens

Preparation Time: 10 minutes
Cooking Time: 10 minutes
Servings: 4

Ingredients:

- 8 cups collard greens, sliced
- 1 onion, chopped
- 6 cloves garlic, chopped
- Salt and pepper to taste
- ¼ cup water
- 1 teaspoon crushed red pepper
- 2 bay leaves
- 1 teaspoon dried thyme

Method:

1. Add all ingredients to the Ninja Foodi.
2. Mix well.
3. Seal the pot.
4. Cook on high for 4 minutes.
5. Release pressure naturally.

Serving Suggestions: Drizzle with vinegar and hot sauce before serving.

Preparation & Cooking Tips: You can also use other leafy greens for this recipe.

Butternut Squash Soup

Preparation Time: 5 minutes
Cooking Time: 30 minutes
Servings: 4

Ingredients:

- 4 cups butternut squash, sliced into cubes
- 1 cup onion, chopped
- 1 tablespoon ginger, minced
- 1 tablespoon garlic, minced
- Salt and pepper to taste
- 1 teaspoon turmeric
- 13 oz. coconut milk
- 1 cup water

Method:

1. Mix all the ingredients in the Ninja Foodi.
2. Lock the lid in place.
3. Cook on high for 8 minutes.
4. Release pressure naturally.
5. Transfer contents of pot to your food processor.
6. Pulse until smooth.

Serving Suggestions: Sprinkle with nutmeg.

Preparation & Cooking Tips: Make big batch of soup and freeze. Reheat for later use.

Kale & Cauliflower Soup

Preparation Time: 10 minutes
Cooking Time: 10 minutes
Servings: 6

Ingredients:

- 1 cup onion, chopped
- 6 cloves garlic, minced
- 12 oz. cauliflower florets
- 12 oz. kale
- 3 cups water
- Salt and pepper to taste
- ½ cup heavy whipping cream

Method:

1. Combine all the ingredients except cream in the Ninja Foodi.
2. Seal the pot.
3. Cook on high for 5 minutes.
4. Release pressure quickly.
5. Let cool.
6. Transfer contents of pot to food processor.
7. Pulse until smooth.
8. Put mixture back to the pot.
9. Set it to sauté.
10. Stir in cream.
11. Heat for 5 minutes.
12. Season with salt and pepper.

Serving Suggestions: Stir in Parmesan cheese.

Preparation & Cooking Tips: You can also use coconut milk for this recipe.

Spicy Cauliflower Soup

Preparation Time: 10 minutes
Cooking Time: 5 minutes
Servings: 4

Ingredients:

- 2 cups cauliflower florets
- 1 ½ cups water
- 1 onion, chopped
- 1 cup carrots, sliced
- 1 cup canned tomatoes
- 1 chili red pepper, chopped
- Salt to taste
- 1 teaspoon turmeric

Method:

1. Add all ingredients to your Ninja Foodi.
2. Seal the pot.
3. Cook on low for 5 minutes.
4. Release pressure quickly.
5. Stir and serve.

Serving Suggestions: Serve with keto bread.

Preparation & Cooking Tips: You can also use cayenne pepper to spice up the soup.

Chapter 8: Fish and Seafood

Spicy Fish Stew

Preparation Time: X minutes
Cooking Time: X minutes
Servings: 2

Ingredients:

- 1 lb. cod fillet
- 1 tablespoon lime juice
- 1 tablespoon olive oil
- 1 jalapeno pepper, seeded and sliced
- 1 onion, sliced
- 1 chili red pepper, chopped
- 2 cloves garlic, minced
- 2 cups tomatoes, chopped
- 1 teaspoon paprika
- 2 cups chicken broth
- 15 oz. coconut milk
- Salt and pepper to taste

Method:

1. Coat fish with lime juice.
2. Cover and marinate for 15 minutes.
3. Add oil to the Ninja Foodi.
4. Set it to sauté.
5. Cook onions and chili pepper for 3 minutes.
6. Stir in garlic and cook for 1 minute.
7. Add the rest of the ingredients.
8. Seal the pot.
9. Cook on high for 5 minutes.

Serving Suggestions: Garnish with cilantro.

Preparation & Cooking Tips: You can also use other white fish fillet for this recipe.

Salmon & Asparagus

Preparation Time: 10 minutes
Cooking Time: 10 minutes
Servings: 4

Ingredients:

- 1 cup water
- 1 clove garlic, crushed
- 5 sprigs dill, chopped
- 1 lb. salmon fillet
- 1 tablespoon butter
- Salt to taste
- ½ teaspoon dried dill
- 1 teaspoon garlic powder
- 6 lemon slices
- 1 cup asparagus, trimmed, sliced and steamed

Method:

1. Pour water into the Ninja Foodi.
2. Add garlic and dill to the water.
3. Place the steamer inside the pot.
4. Add the salmon on top of the steamer.
5. Spread salmon with butter, and
6. Season with the salt, dried dill and garlic powder.
7. Top with lemon slices.
8. Seal the pot.
9. Cook on high for 4 minutes.
10. Release pressure quickly.
11. Serve with steamed asparagus.

Serving Suggestions: Serve with creamy sauce and capers.

Preparation & Cooking Tips: You can also steam the asparagus in the Ninja Foodi.

Crab Legs

Preparation Time: 3 minutes
Cooking Time: 3 minutes
Servings: 4

Ingredients:

- 2 lb. crab legs
- 1 cup water
- ¼ cup butter

Method:

1. Add water to the Ninja Foodi.
2. Place the steamer inside.
3. Place the crab legs on top of the steamer.
4. Seal the pot.
5. Cook on high for 3 minutes.
6. Release pressure quickly.
7. Serve with butter.

Serving Suggestions: Garnish with lemon slices.

Preparation & Cooking Tips: Use grass-fed butter or herbed butter.

Fish Curry

Preparation Time: 10 minutes
Cooking Time: 10 minutes
Servings: 4

Ingredients:

- 2 tablespoons coconut oil
- 10 curry leaves
- 1 cup onion, chopped
- 1 tablespoon ginger, minced
- 1 chili pepper, sliced
- 1 tablespoon garlic, minced
- 1 cup tomato, chopped
- Salt and pepper to taste
- ½ teaspoon turmeric powder
- ¼ teaspoon cumin powder
- 1 teaspoon coriander powder
- 1 ½ lb. cod fillet
- 2 tablespoons water
- 1 cup coconut milk
- 1 teaspoon lime juice

Method:

1. Set your Ninja Foodi to sauté.
2. Add coconut oil and cook curry leaves for 30 seconds.
3. Stir in onion, ginger, chili pepper and garlic.
4. Cook for 2 minutes.
5. Add tomatoes and cook for 3 minutes.
6. Season with salt, pepper and spices.
7. Cook while stirring for 30 seconds.
8. Add fish, water and coconut milk.
9. Lock the lid in place.
10. Cook on high for 2 minutes.
11. Release pressure quickly.

12. Stir in lime juice before serving.

Serving Suggestions: Garnish with fresh tomato slices.

Preparation & Cooking Tips: You can also use cod fillet for this recipe.

Fish with Black Bean & Ginger

Preparation Time: 2 hours and 10 minutes
Cooking Time: 10 minutes
Servings: 4

Ingredients:

- 2 tablespoons rice wine
- 3 tablespoons soy sauce
- 1 tablespoon black bean paste
- 1 clove garlic, minced
- 1 lb. white fish fillet
- 1 cup water

Method:

1. In a bowl, mix all the ingredients except fish and water.
2. Add fish and cover.
3. Marinate in the refrigerator for 2 hours.
4. Add water to the Ninja Foodi.
5. Place steamer inside.
6. Add fish on top of steamer.
7. Brush with marinade.
8. Seal the pot.
9. Cook on low for 2 minutes.
10. Release pressure quickly.

Serving Suggestions: Garnish with chopped scallions.

Preparation & Cooking Tips: You can also serve steamed fish with vegetables.

Fish Saag

Preparation Time: 10 minutes
Cooking Time: 5 minutes
Servings: 4

Ingredients:

Sauce

- ½ cup coconut milk
- 2 onions, chopped
- 1 tablespoon garlic, minced
- 1 tablespoon ginger, minced
- 1 cup tomatoes, chopped
- 1 teaspoon turmeric
- 1 teaspoon garam masala
- 1 teaspoon cayenne pepper
- 2 cups spinach
- ¼ cup water
- Salt to taste

Fish

- 1 lb. haddock fillet, sliced into cubes
- 1 teaspoon turmeric
- Salt to taste
- 1 cup water

Method:

1. Combine the sauce ingredients in the Ninja Foodi.
2. Set it to sauté.
3. Cook while stirring for 10 to 15 minutes.
4. Transfer to a bowl and set aside.
5. Season fish with turmeric and salt.
6. Add to a steamer.
7. Place steamer inside the Ninja Foodi.
8. Pour in water.

9. Seal the pot.
10. Cook on high for 3 minutes.
11. Release pressure naturally.
12. Pour sauce over the fish and serve.

Serving Suggestions: Serve with cauliflower rice.

Preparation & Cooking Tips: You can also use other white fish fillet for this recipe.

Creamy Shrimp

Preparation Time: 5 minutes
Cooking Time: 10 minutes
Servings: 6

Ingredients:

- 2 tablespoons butter
- 1 lb. shrimp, peeled and deveined
- 4 cloves garlic, minced
- ½ teaspoons red pepper flakes
- ½ teaspoon smoked paprika
- 1 cup chicken broth
- Salt and pepper to taste
- ½ cup Parmesan cheese
- ½ cup half and half

Method:

1. Set the Ninja Foodi to sauté.
2. Add butter.
3. Cook garlic and crushed red pepper for 2 minutes.
4. Stir in the rest of the ingredients except cheese and half and half.
5. Seal the pot.
6. Cook on high for 2 minutes.
7. Release pressure quickly.
8. Stir in cheese and half and half before serving.

Serving Suggestions: Garnish with chopped chives.

Preparation & Cooking Tips: You can also use frozen shrimp for this recipe.

Garlic Shrimp

Preparation Time: 10 minutes
Cooking Time: 5 minutes
Servings: 4

Ingredients:

- 3 tablespoons butter
- 2 tablespoons olive oil
- 6 cloves garlic, minced
- 1 cup chicken broth
- ¼ cup white wine
- 2 lb. shrimp, peeled and deveined
- 1 ½ tablespoons lemon juice
- Salt and pepper to taste

Method:

1. Choose sauté function in the Ninja Foodi.
2. Add butter and olive oil.
3. Cook garlic for 3 minutes.
4. Pour in broth and wine.
5. Stir in shrimp.
6. Cover the pot.
7. Cook on high for 1 minute.
8. Release pressure naturally.
9. Stir in the lemon juice.
10. Season with salt and pepper.

Serving Suggestions: Garnish with chopped parsley.

Preparation & Cooking Tips: You can also use frozen peeled shrimp to save time.

Lemon Herbed Salmon

Preparation Time: 5 minutes
Cooking Time: 3 minutes
Servings: 4

Ingredients:

- ¾ cup water
- 1 lb. salmon fillets
- 3 teaspoons ghee
- Salt and pepper to taste
- 2 sprigs tarragon
- 2 sprigs dill
- 6 lemon slices

Method:

1. Add water to the Ninja Foodi.
2. Place the steamer inside.
3. Brush both sides of salmon with ghee.
4. Sprinkle with salt and pepper.
5. Top with herb sprigs and lemon slices.
6. Seal the pot.
7. Cook on high for 3 minutes.
8. Release pressure naturally.

Serving Suggestions: Discard herb sprigs before serving.

Preparation & Cooking Tips: Use salmon fillets 1 inch thick for this recipe.

Shrimp & Broccoli

Preparation Time: 10 minutes
Cooking Time: 2 minutes
Servings: 4

Ingredients:

- 4 cups broccoli florets
- 1 lb. shrimp, peeled and deveined
- 2 tablespoons ginger, grated
- 2 cloves garlic, minced
- 2 tablespoons oyster sauce
- ¼ cup soy sauce
- 1 teaspoon rice wine vinegar
- 2 teaspoons brown sugar

Method:

1. Combine all the ingredients in the Ninja Foodi.
2. Lock the lid in place.
3. Cook on high for 2 minutes.
4. Release pressure quickly.

Serving Suggestions: Garnish with white sesame seeds.

Preparation & Cooking Tips: You can also serve this dish with cauliflower rice.

Chapter 9: Poultry

Chicken With Garlic Butter

Preparation Time: 10 minutes
Cooking Time: 40 minutes
Servings: 4

Ingredients:

- 10 cloves garlic, minced
- ¼ cup butter
- 4 chicken breasts, chopped
- Salt to taste

Method:

1. Add all the ingredients to your Ninja Foodi.
2. Lock the lid in place.
3. Cook on high for 40 minutes.
4. Release pressure naturally.

Serving Suggestions: Serve with cauliflower rice.

Preparation & Cooking Tips: You can also cook the chicken breast fillet whole.

Shredded Chicken

Preparation Time: 5 minutes
Cooking Time: 20 minutes
Servings: 8

Ingredients:

- 4 lb. chicken breast fillet
- ½ cup chicken broth
- Salt and pepper to taste

Method:

1. Combine the ingredients in the Ninja Foodi.
2. Seal the pot.
3. Cook on high for 20 minutes.
4. Release pressure quickly.
5. Shred the chicken.

Serving Suggestions: Serve with cauliflower rice or steamed vegetables.

Preparation & Cooking Tips: You can use shredded chicken for your sandwich. Make sure to use keto bread.

Coconut Lemon Turkey

Preparation Time: 10 minutes
Cooking Time: 4 hours
Servings: 6

Ingredients:

- 3 cups coconut milk
- ¼ cup lemon juice
- 1 tablespoon curry powder
- Salt to taste
- 1 teaspoon turmeric
- 6 turkey breasts

Method:

1. Set your Ninja Foodi to slow cook.
2. Combine all ingredients in the pot.
3. Seal the pot.
4. Cook for 4 hours.

Serving Suggestions: Garnish with lemon wedges.

Preparation & Cooking Tips: You can also use chicken for this recipe.

Butter Chicken

Preparation Time: X minutes
Cooking Time: X minutes
Servings: 5

Ingredients:

- 2 tablespoons oil
- 1 onion, diced
- 1 teaspoon ginger, minced
- 5 cloves garlic, minced
- 1 ½ lb. chicken thigh fillets, sliced into cubes
- 1 teaspoon paprika
- 1 teaspoon garam masala
- 1 teaspoon coriander powder
- 1 teaspoon turmeric
- ¼ teaspoon ground cumin
- ¼ teaspoon cayenne
- Salt and pepper to taste
- 15 oz. tomato sauce

Method:

1. Set the Ninja Foodi to sauté.
2. Add the oil and cook onions for 5 minutes, stirring.
3. Stir in the ginger, garlic and chicken.
4. Cook for 7 minutes.
5. Add all the spices.
6. Mix well.
7. Pour in tomato sauce.
8. Seal the pot.
9. Cook on high for 8 minutes.
10. Release pressure quickly.

Serving Suggestions: Garnish with fresh cilantro.

Preparation & Cooking Tips: You can also stir in a cup of coconut milk before serving.

Chicken Tikka Masala

Preparation Time: 10 minutes
Cooking Time: 25 minutes
Servings: 6

Ingredients:

- 1 onion, chopped
- 1 red bell pepper, chopped
- 2 tablespoons butter
- 1 teaspoon ginger, grated
- 3 cloves garlic, minced
- Salt to taste
- 2 teaspoons garam masala
- 1 teaspoon turmeric
- 1 teaspoon coriander
- 1 teaspoon cumin
- ¼ teaspoon cayenne pepper
- 15 oz. canned tomatoes
- ½ cup coconut milk
- 2 lb. chicken breast fillet, sliced into cubes

Method:

1. Select sauté function in your Ninja Foodi.
2. Cook onion and bell pepper in butter for 4 minutes.
3. Stir in the ginger, garlic, salt and spices.
4. Cook while stirring for 1 minute.
5. Add coconut milk and tomatoes.
6. Top with the chicken.
7. Cook on high for 15 minutes.
8. Release pressure naturally.
9. Shred chicken and put shredded chicken back to the pot.
10. Puree sauce mixture using a food processor.
11. Serve chicken with pureed sauce.

Serving Suggestions: Serve with fresh green salad.

Preparation & Cooking Tips: Add more cayenne pepper for extra spiciness.

Turkey Buffalo Meatballs

Preparation Time: 10 minutes
Cooking Time: 20 minutes
Servings: 6

Ingredients:

Meatball

- 1 ½ lb. ground turkey
- 2 cloves garlic, minced
- ¾ cup almond meal
- 1 teaspoon salt

Sauce

- 2 tablespoons ghee
- 4 tablespoons butter
- 6 tablespoons hot sauce

Method:

1. Mix all meatball ingredients in a bowl.
2. Form meatballs from this mixture.
3. Set Ninja Foodi to sauté.
4. Add ghee.
5. Cook meatballs until browned on all sides.
6. Combine butter and hot sauce in a bowl.
7. Pour into the pot.
8. Close the pot.
9. Cook on high for 3 minutes.
10. Release pressure naturally.

Serving Suggestions: Serve with zucchini noodles or cauliflower rice.

Preparation & Cooking Tips: You can also add chopped chives in the meatball.

Chicken Adobo

Preparation Time: 15 minutes
Cooking Time: 30 minutes
Servings: 4

Ingredients:

- 1 tablespoon oil
- 2 chicken thigh fillets, sliced into strips
- 1 onion, sliced
- 5 cloves garlic, minced
- ¼ cup vinegar
- ½ cup soy sauce
- 3 bay leaves
- Salt and pepper to taste

Method:

1. Set Ninja Foodi to sauté.
2. Add oil and brown chicken strips.
3. Add the rest of the ingredients.
4. Seal the pot.
5. Cook on high for 10 minutes.
6. Release pressure quickly.
7. Press sauté mode and cook until sauce has thickened.

Serving Suggestions: Discard bay leaves before serving.

Preparation & Cooking Tips: You can also season chicken with cayenne pepper.

Rosemary Chicken

Preparation Time: 10 minutes
Cooking Time: 10 minutes
Servings: 4

Ingredients:

- 1 cup water
- 4 chicken breast fillets
- Salt and pepper to taste
- 8 sprigs rosemary
- 8 slices lemon

Method:

1. Add water to your Ninja Foodi.
2. Place steamer inside.
3. Season chicken with salt and pepper.
4. Add to the steamer.
5. Top with rosemary sprigs and lemon slices.
6. Seal the pot.
7. Cook on high for 10 minutes.
8. Release pressure naturally.

Serving Suggestions: Discard herb sprigs before serving.

Preparation & Cooking Tips: You can also drizzle chicken with lemon juice before cooking.

Savory Turkey Breast

Preparation Time: 10 minutes
Cooking Time: 30 minutes
Servings: 8

Ingredients:

- 1 packet onion soup mix
- 6 turkey breast fillets
- 1 onion, sliced
- 2 stalks celery, sliced
- 1 cup chicken broth
- 2 tablespoons water mixed with 1 tablespoon cornstarch

Method:

1. Season turkey with onion soup mix.
2. Add to Ninja Foodi.
3. Top turkey with onion and celery.
4. Pour chicken broth around the turkey.
5. Cover the pot.
6. Cook on low for 30 minutes.
7. Release pressure naturally.
8. Set Ninja Foodi to sauté.
9. Add cornstarch mixture to the cooking liquid.
10. Cook until sauce has thickened.

Serving Suggestions: Garnish with chopped parsley.

Preparation & Cooking Tips: You can also add pepper to the sauce.

Chicken Barbecue

Preparation Time: 5 minutes
Cooking Time: 20 minutes
Servings: 8

Ingredients:

- 2 lb. chicken thigh fillets
- Salt and pepper to taste
- 1 teaspoon ground paprika
- 3 cups barbecue sauce

Method:

1. Season chicken with salt, pepper and paprika.
2. Add to the Ninja Foodi.
3. Pour in the sauce.
4. Cover the pot.
5. Cook on high for 20 minutes.
6. Release pressure naturally.

Serving Suggestions: Pour sauce over the chicken before serving.

Preparation & Cooking Tips: You can also make your own barbecue sauce by mixing ketchup, honey and soy sauce.

Chapter 10: Beef, Pork & Lamb

Chili Lime Steak

Preparation Time: 10 minutes
Cooking Time: 10 minutes
Servings: 4

Ingredients:

- 1 tablespoon olive oil
- 1 teaspoon garlic, minced
- 1 ½ lb. steak strips
- 2 teaspoons lime juice
- ½ teaspoon chili powder
- 1 tablespoon water
- Salt and pepper to taste

Method:

1. Add olive oil to Ninja Foodi.
2. Cook garlic for 2 minutes, stirring frequently.
3. Add the rest of the ingredients.
4. Mix well.
5. Seal the pot.
6. Cook on high for 10 minutes.
7. Release pressure quickly.

Serving Suggestions: Serve with avocado cubes.

Preparation & Cooking Tips: You can also slice steak into cubes.

Beef Short Ribs

Preparation Time: 10 minutes
Cooking Time: 45 minutes
Servings: 4

Ingredients:

- 1 onion, chopped
- 2 lb. beef short ribs
- Salt to taste
- 3 tablespoons tamari sauce
- 2 tablespoons white wine
- 1 cup water

Method:

1. Add all ingredients to the Ninja Foodi.
2. Press meat or stew function and cook for 45 minutes.
3. Or you can pressure cook on high for 30 minutes.

Serving Suggestions: Pour sauce over the ribs before serving.

Preparation & Cooking Tips: You can also add curry powder and star anise to the cooking liquid.

Mexican Beef

Preparation Time: 15 minutes
Cooking Time: 35 minutes
Servings: 6

Ingredients:

- 2 ½ lb. beef brisket, sliced into cubes
- Salt to taste
- 1 tablespoon chili powder
- 1 tablespoon oil
- 1 onion, sliced
- 6 cloves garlic, peeled and crushed
- 1 tablespoon tomato paste
- ½ cup tomato salsa
- ½ cup beef broth
- ½ teaspoon fish sauce
- Pepper to taste

Method:

1. Season beef with salt and chili powder.
2. Set Ninja Foodi to sauté.
3. Add oil to the pot.
4. Cook onion for 2 minutes.
5. Stir in garlic and tomato paste.
6. Cook for 1 minute.
7. Add beef and the rest of the ingredients.
8. Seal the pot.
9. Cook on high for 35 minutes.
10. Release pressure naturally.
11. Pour sauce over the beef and serve.

Serving Suggestions: Serve with thinly sliced radish.

Preparation & Cooking Tips: Use roasted salsa for best results.

Braised Beef

Preparation Time: 15 minutes
Cooking Time: 40 minutes
Servings: 8

Ingredients:

- 3 lb. beef stew meat, sliced into cubes
- 1 tablespoon cumin
- 1 tablespoon chili powder
- Red pepper flakes
- Salt to taste
- 2 tablespoons olive oil
- 1 tablespoon lime juice
- 1 cup beef broth
- 3 oz. tomato paste
- 1 onion, chopped

Method:

1. Season beef with cumin, chili powder, red pepper flakes and salt.
2. Add oil to the Ninja Foodi.
3. Set it to sauté.
4. Cook beef until browned on all sides.
5. Add the rest of the ingredients.
6. Seal the pot.
7. Cook on high for 35 minutes.
8. Release pressure naturally.

Serving Suggestions: Serve with green salad or cauliflower rice.

Preparation & Cooking Tips: Omit red pepper if you don't want your braised beef spicy.

Beef Stroganoff

Preparation Time: 10 minutes
Cooking Time: 30 minutes
Servings: 4

Ingredients:

- 1 tablespoon coconut oil
- 1 onion, chopped
- 1 lb. ground beef
- 2 tablespoons white wine vinegar
- 1 cup chicken broth
- 1 teaspoon dried parsley
- 1 cup shiitake mushrooms
- Salt and pepper to taste

Method:

1. Set your Ninja Foodi to sauté.
2. Add coconut oil.
3. Cook onion for 1 minute, stirring often.
4. Add ground beef and cook until browned.
5. Add the rest of the ingredients.
6. Secure the lid.
7. Cook on high for 25 minutes.
8. Release pressure naturally.

Serving Suggestions: Serve on top of spaghetti squash.

Preparation & Cooking Tips: You can also add cream or coconut milk to the mixture.

Pot Roast with Gravy

Preparation Time: 10 minutes
Cooking Time: 1 hour
Servings: 6

Ingredients:

- 4 lb. chuck roast, sliced into 4
- Salt and pepper to taste
- 1 ½ cups beef broth
- 2 tablespoons vinegar
- 2 teaspoons fish sauce
- 1 sprig rosemary
- 4 sprigs thyme
- 6 cloves garlic, peeled

Method:

1. Sprinkle beef with salt and pepper.
2. Add to the Ninja Foodi.
3. Stir in the rest of the ingredients.
4. Cover the pot.
5. Cook on high for 1 hour.
6. Release pressure naturally.
7. Discard herb sprigs.
8. Transfer cooking liquid to food processor.
9. Puree the sauce.
10. Serve pot roast with gravy.

Serving Suggestions: Serve with mashed cauliflower.

Preparation & Cooking Tips: Use balsamic vinegar for better results.

Pork Carnitas

Preparation Time: 8 hours and 10 minutes
Cooking Time: 1 hour
Servings: 4

Ingredients:

Rub

- 1/2 teaspoon ground coriander
- 1 teaspoon onion salt
- 1 teaspoon cayenne pepper
- 1 tablespoon cocoa powder
- 1 teaspoon garlic powder
- 1 teaspoon ground cumin
- 2 teaspoons dried oregano
- Salt and pepper to taste

Pork

- 3 lb. pork shoulder
- 2 tablespoons olive oil
- 3 cups water

Method:

1. Combine rub ingredients in a bowl.
2. Massage mixture on all sides of pork.
3. Cover and refrigerate for 8 hours.
4. Set the Ninja Foodi to sauté.
5. Pour in the oil.
6. Add pork to the pot.
7. Cook until browned on all sides.
8. Pour in water.
9. Secure the lid.
10. Cook on high pressure for 45 minutes.
11. Release pressure naturally.
12. Let cool.

13. Shred the pork with 2 forks.
14. Put shredded pork to the pot.
15. Press sauté.
16. Cook for 5 minutes.

Serving Suggestions: Wrap shredded pork in lettuce before serving.

Preparation & Cooking Tips: If using in lettuce rolls, add radish and carrot strips or chopped tomatoes.

Vietnamese Pork Tenderloin

Preparation Time: 2 hours and 10 minutes
Cooking Time: 10 minutes
Servings: 6

Ingredients:

Marinade

- 1 cup chicken stock
- ½ teaspoon garlic, minced
- ½ teaspoon ginger, minced
- ½ lemongrass, minced
- 1 shallot, minced
- 1 tablespoon soy sauce
- 1 tablespoon fish sauce
- 2 teaspoons brown sugar
- ¼ teaspoon red pepper flakes
- Salt to taste

Pork

- 2 ½ lb. pork tenderloin
- 1 tablespoon coconut oil

Method:

1. Mix marinade ingredients in a bowl.
2. Reserve half and refrigerate.
3. Add pork tenderloin to the remaining mixture.
4. Marinate for 2 hours.
5. Set the Ninja Foodi to sauté.
6. Pour oil to the pot.
7. Cook pork tenderloin for 3 minutes or until brown on all sides.
8. Add reserved sauce to the pot.
9. Seal the pot.
10. Cook on high for 7 minutes.
11. Release pressure quickly.

Serving Suggestions: Garnish with lemon zest and lemon slices.

Preparation & Cooking Tips: You can also use beef for this recipe.

Jamaican Jerk Pork Roast

Preparation Time: 15 minutes
Cooking Time: 50 minutes
Servings: 4

Ingredients:

- 4 lb. pork shoulder
- ¼ cup Jamaican Jerk spice mixture
- 1 tablespoon olive oil
- ½ cup beef broth

Method:

1. Coat the pork shoulder with oil.
2. Rub with seasoning mixture.
3. Press sauté setting in the Ninja Foodi.
4. Pour the olive oil to the pot.
5. Cook the pork until browned on all sides.
6. Pour in the broth.
7. Secure the lid.
8. Cook on high for 45 minutes.
9. Shred the pork.

Serving Suggestions: Wrap in lettuce or use as topping for tacos.

Preparation & Cooking Tips: You can also add cayenne pepper to the spice blend.

Pork Stew

Preparation Time: 15 minutes
Cooking Time: 50 minutes
Servings: 4

Ingredients:

- 2 tablespoons avocado oil
- 4 lb. pork tenderloin, sliced into cubes
- Salt to taste
- 1 onion, chopped
- 6 cloves garlic, minced
- 1 leek, chopped
- 8 oz. mushrooms
- 1 ½ cups pork broth
- 2 tablespoons lemon juice

Method:

1. Set the Ninja Foodi to sauté.
2. Add avocado oil.
3. Cook pork cubes until browned on all sides.
4. Season with salt.
5. Add the onion, garlic and leeks.
6. Cook for 2 minutes, stirring often.
7. Stir in the rest of the ingredients except lemon juice.
8. Seal the pot.
9. Cook on high for 45 minutes.

Serving Suggestions: Serve with keto bread.

Preparation & Cooking Tips: You can make a big batch and freeze for later use.

Pork Belly with Cauliflower Rice

Preparation Time: 15 minutes
Cooking Time: 15 minutes
Servings: 4

Ingredients:

- 1 lb. pork belly, cooked and sliced into cubes
- ½ cup cilantro, divided
- 1 tablespoon oil
- ½ cup bone broth
- 4 cups cauliflower rice
- ½ onion, sliced
- 3 cloves garlic, sliced
- 2 green onions, sliced
- 1 tablespoon lime juice
- 1 tablespoon cumin
- 1 tablespoon oregano
- 1 teaspoon turmeric
- Salt to taste

Method:

1. Add pork, half of cilantro and the rest of the ingredients to your Ninja Foodi.
2. Mix well.
3. Lock the lid in place.
4. Cook on high for 15 minutes.
5. Release pressure naturally.
6. Transfer to serving bowls.
7. Sprinkle with remaining cilantro.

Serving Suggestions: Serve with steamed or stir-fried veggies.

Preparation & Cooking Tips: You can also slow cook this dish for 3 to 4 hours in your Ninja Foodi.

Pork Taco Bowl

Preparation Time: 20 minutes
Cooking Time: 1 hour
Servings: 6

Ingredients:

- 2 lb. pork sirloin roast, sliced into strips
- Salt and pepper to taste
- 2 teaspoons garlic powder
- 2 teaspoons ground cumin
- 1 tablespoon olive oil
- 16 oz. tomato salsa
- Cauliflower rice

Method:

1. Season pork with salt, pepper, garlic powder and cumin.
2. Set Ninja Foodi to sauté.
3. Add oil and cook pork strips until browned.
4. Add the salsa.
5. Seal the pot.
6. Cook on high for 45 minutes.
7. Release pressure naturally.
8. Serve in bowls with cauliflower rice.

Serving Suggestions: Serve with sour cream, chopped avocado and grated Mexican cheese.

Preparation & Cooking Tips: You can also slow cook the pork in your Ninja Foodi for 3 to 4 hours.

Lamb Stew

Preparation Time: 15 minutes
Cooking Time: 35 minutes
Servings: 6

Ingredients:

- 1 yellow onion, sliced into wedges
- 6 cloves garlic, sliced
- 2 lb. lamb stew meat
- 3 carrots, sliced into rounds,
- 1 acorn squash, sliced into cubes
- 1 bay leaf
- 2 sprigs rosemary
- 1 cup beef broth
- Salt to taste

Method:

1. Add all ingredients to your Ninja Foodi.
2. Secure the lid.
3. Cook on high for 35 minutes.
4. Release pressure naturally.
5. Serve stew in bowls.

Serving Suggestions: Discard herb sprigs before serving.

Preparation & Cooking Tips: You can also use beef or goat meat for this recipe.

Coconut Lamb Shanks

Preparation Time: 10 minutes
Cooking Time: 50 minutes
Servings: 2

Ingredients:

Spice mixture

- 1 tablespoon smoked paprika
- 1 tablespoon ground coriander
- 1 tablespoon dried onion flakes
- 1 teaspoon garam masala
- 1 tablespoon ground cumin
- Salt and pepper to taste

Lamb

- 2 lamb shanks
- 2 tablespoons avocado oil
- 1 teaspoon garlic, minced
- 1 tablespoon ginger, minced
- 1 tablespoon tomato paste
- ½ cup water
- ¼ cup coconut milk

Method:

1. Combine spice mixture ingredients in a bowl.
2. Massage lamb shanks with this mixture.
3. Choose sauté setting in your Ninja Foodi.
4. Add oil to the pot.
5. Cook the lamb for 5 minutes.
6. Stir in the garlic, ginger and tomato paste.
7. Add remaining spice mixture.
8. Cook while stirring for 2 minutes.
9. Pour in water and coconut milk.
10. Seal the pot.

11. Cook on high for 45 minutes.

12. Release pressure naturally.

Serving Suggestions: Garnish with fresh cilantro.

Preparation & Cooking Tips: You can add cornstarch mixed with water to the cooking liquid to thicken the sauce.

Lamb Curry

Preparation Time: 15 minutes
Cooking Time: 20 minutes
Servings: 4

Ingredients:

- 1 tablespoon butter
- 1 onion, diced
- 2 tablespoons ginger, minced
- 2 cloves garlic, crushed and minced
- 1 lb. lamb stew meat
- 2 cups canned tomatoes
- 3 cloves
- 1 teaspoon ground cardamom
- 2 teaspoons ground coriander
- 1 tablespoon garam masala
- 1 teaspoon turmeric
- 2 teaspoon cumin
- Salt to taste
- 1 red bell pepper, chopped
- 1 zucchini, chopped
- 2 cups kale, sliced

Method:

1. Add the butter to the Ninja Foodi.
2. Set it to sauté.
3. Cook onion, ginger and garlic for 1 minute, stirring often.
4. Add lamb and cook until browned.
5. Stir in canned tomatoes and the rest of the ingredients except vegetables.
6. Lock the lid in place.
7. Cook on high for 20 minutes.
8. Release pressure naturally.
9. Set Ninja Foodi back to sauté.
10. Add vegetables.

11. Cook until tender.

Serving Suggestions: Garnish with cilantro.

Preparation & Cooking Tips: You can also add carrots to this mixture.

Rosemary Lamb

Preparation Time: 10 minutes
Cooking Time: 2 hours
Servings: 4

Ingredients:

- 1 tablespoon butter
- 1 onion, chopped
- 2 stalks celery, chopped
- 1 carrot, chopped
- 1 cup red wine
- 1 tablespoon tomato paste
- 2 cups beef stock
- 1 tablespoon rosemary, chopped
- 4 lamb shanks
- 1 bay leaf
- Salt and pepper to taste

Method:

1. Set Ninja Foodi to sauté.
2. Add butter and cook onion, celery and carrot for 2 minutes.
3. Pour in wine.
4. Cook until reduced by half.
5. Stir in tomato paste and remaining ingredients.
6. Secure the lid.
7. Cook on high for 2 hours.

Serving Suggestions: Serve with mashed cauliflower.

Preparation & Cooking Tips: You can also use bone broth in place of beef stock.

Chapter 11: Desserts

Blueberry Cupcake

Preparation Time: X minutes
Cooking Time: X minutes
Servings: 8

Ingredients:

- 4 ½ tablespoon erythritol sweetener
- 1 ½ tablespoon golden flaxseed meal
- 1/3 cup coconut flour
- ¼ teaspoon baking soda
- 1 teaspoon baking powder
- ⅛ teaspoon salt
- 2 eggs, beaten
- 1/3 cup almond milk (unsweetened)
- 1 teaspoon vanilla extract
- 1 ½ tablespoons butter
- 1/3 cup fresh blueberries
- 1 cup water

Method:

1. In a bowl, mix sweetener, flaxseed meal, coconut flour, baking soda, baking powder and salt.
2. In another bowl, combine the remaining ingredients except blueberries and water.
3. Add first bowl to the second.
4. Fold in blueberries.
5. Pour water into the Ninja Foodi.
6. Pour cupcake molds with mixture.
7. Cover with foil.
8. Add steamer to the pot.
9. Place cupcake molds on top of the steamer.
10. Seal the pot.
11. Cook on high for 20 minutes.

12. Release pressure naturally.

Serving Suggestions: Let cool before serving.

Preparation & Cooking Tips: You can also use other berries for this recipe.

Pumpkin Pie

Preparation Time: 10 minutes
Cooking Time: 30 minutes
Servings: 6

Ingredients:

- 15 oz. pumpkin puree
- 2 eggs, beaten
- ¾ cup erythritol sweetener
- ½ cup heavy whipping cream
- 1 teaspoon vanilla extract
- 1 teaspoon pumpkin pie spice
- 1 ½ cups water

Method:

1. Combine all ingredients except water in a bowl.
2. Pour mixture into a small baking pan.
3. Cover with foil.
4. Add steamer inside your Ninja Foodi.
5. Place the pan on top of the steamer.
6. Cook on high for 20 minutes.
7. Release pressure naturally.

Serving Suggestions: Serve with whipped cream.

Preparation & Cooking Tips: Refrigerate for 8 hours before serving.

Molten Brownie Cups

Preparation Time: 15 minutes
Cooking Time: 10 minutes
Servings: 4

Ingredients:

- Cooking spray
- 6 tablespoons butter
- 2/3 cup keto-friendly chocolate chips
- 3 eggs, beaten
- ⅔ cup keto sweetener
- 3 ½ tablespoons almond flour
- 1 teaspoon vanilla extract
- 1 ¾ cups water

Method:

1. Spray ramekins with oil.
2. Set your Ninja Foodi to sauté.
3. Add butter and chocolate chips.
4. Heat while stirring until melted.
5. In a bowl, mix the remaining ingredients except water.
6. Add butter mixture to this bowl.
7. Mix well.
8. Pour batter into the ramekins.
9. Add water to the pot.
10. Place a steamer inside.
11. Add the ramekins to the steamer.
12. Seal the pot.
13. Cook on high for 10 minutes.
14. Release pressure quickly.

Serving Suggestions: Top with sugar-free whipping cream.

Preparation & Cooking Tips: You can also add walnuts to the batter.

Coconut Almond Cake

Preparation Time: 10 minutes
Cooking Time: 40 minutes
Servings: 8

Ingredients:

- 2 cups water

Dry ingredients

- 1 cup almond flour
- 1 teaspoon baking powder
- 1/3 cup keto sweetener
- 1 teaspoon apple pie spice
- ½ cup coconut flakes

Wet ingredients

- ¼ cup butter
- 2 eggs, beaten
- ½ cup whipping cream

Method:

1. Combine dry ingredients in a bowl.
2. Add wet ingredients to the bowl one by one.
3. Mix well.
4. Pour into a small baking pan.
5. Cover with foil.
6. Pour water to the Ninja Foodi.
7. Place the steamer inside.
8. Add baking pan on top of steamer.
9. Seal the pot.
10. Cook on high for 40 minutes.
11. Release pressure naturally.

Serving Suggestions: Let cool for 20 minutes before slicing and serving.

Preparation & Cooking Tips: Make sure that you use unsweetened coconut flakes for this recipe.

Cheesecake

Preparation Time: 4 hours and 20 minutes
Cooking Time: 40 minutes
Servings: 8

Ingredients:

- Cooking spray
- 1 teaspoon vegetable oil
- 8 oz. cream cheese
- 1 teaspoon vanilla extract
- 1 teaspoon lemon zest
- 2 eggs
- 2/3 cup keto sweetener
- 1 cup water

Method:

1. Spray your small baking pan with oil.
2. Use a mixer to blend cream cheese and the rest of the ingredients except water.
3. Pour mixture into the baking pan.
4. Cover with foil.
5. Pour water into the Ninja Foodi.
6. Add steamer inside the pot.
7. Place baking pan on top of steamer.
8. Seal the pot.
9. Cook on high for 20 minutes.
10. Release pressure naturally.
11. Let cool.
12. Transfer baking pan to refrigerator.
13. Refrigerate for 4 hours.

Serving Suggestions: Top cheesecake with chopped almonds.

Preparation & Cooking Tips: You can refrigerate the cheesecake longer.

Coconut Pandan Custard

Preparation Time: 5 minutes
Cooking Time: 30 minutes
Servings: 4

Ingredients:

- 1 cup coconut milk
- 3 eggs, beaten
- 1/3 cup keto sweetener
- 3 drops pandan extract
- 2 cups water

Method:

1. Mix all ingredients except water in a heatproof bowl.
2. Cover the bowl with foil.
3. Add water to the Ninja Foodi.
4. Place a steamer inside.
5. Add the bowl to the steamer.
6. Secure the lid.
7. Cook on high for 30 minutes.
8. Release pressure naturally.

Serving Suggestions: Sprinkle top with unsweetened coconut flakes.

Preparation & Cooking Tips: You can use vanilla extract if pandan extract is not available.

Ricotta Lemon Cheesecake

Preparation Time: 10 minutes
Cooking Time: 40 minutes
Servings: 6

Ingredients:

- ¼ cup keto sweetener
- 8 oz. cream cheese
- 1 teaspoon lemon zest
- 1/3 cup ricotta cheese
- ½ teaspoon lemon extract
- ¼ cup lemon juice
- 2 eggs, beaten
- 2 cups water

Method:

1. Add keto sweetener, cream cheese, lemon zest, ricotta cheese, lemon extract and lemon juice to a bowl.
2. Mix well.
3. Stir in eggs.
4. Mix until fully combined.
5. Pour mixture into a small baking pan.
6. Cover the pan with foil.
7. Pour water into your Ninja Foodi.
8. Seal the pot.
9. Cook on high for 30 minutes.
10. Release pressure naturally.
11. Let cool.
12. Refrigerate cake for 8 hours.

Serving Suggestions: Top with sour cream mixed with keto sweetener.

Preparation & Cooking Tips: Use freshly squeezed lemon juice.

Chocolate Cake

Preparation Time: 10 minutes
Cooking Time: 20 minutes
Servings: 6

Ingredients:

- 1 cup almond flour
- ¼ cup cocoa powder (unsweetened)
- 1 teaspoon baking powder
- 2/3 cup keto sweetener
- 1/3 cup whipping cream
- 3 eggs, beaten
- ¼ cup coconut oil
- ¼ cup walnuts, chopped
- 2 cups water

Method:

1. Combine all ingredients except water in a bowl.
2. Transfer mixture to a small baking pan.
3. Cover with foil.
4. Add water to the Ninja Foodi.
5. Place the steamer inside.
6. Secure the lid.
7. Cook on high for 20 minutes.
8. Release pressure naturally.

Serving Suggestions: Sprinkle with chopped walnuts on top.

Preparation & Cooking Tips: Use an electric mixer to mix the ingredients more conveniently.

Almond Cake

Preparation Time: 10 minutes
Cooking Time: 40 minutes
Servings: 8

Ingredients:

- 2 cups water

Dry ingredients

- 1 cup almond flour
- 1 teaspoon apple pie spice
- 1 teaspoon baking powder
- 1/3 cup sweetener

Wet ingredients

- ¼ cup butter
- 2 eggs, beaten
- ½ cup heavy whipping cream

Method:

1. Combine dry ingredients in a bowl.
2. Add wet ingredients to this bowl.
3. Transfer mixture to a baking pan.
4. Cover with foil.
5. Place steamer inside the Ninja Foodi.
6. Pour in water.
7. Add baking pan to the steamer.
8. Seal the pot.
9. Cook on high for 10 minutes.
10. Release pressure naturally.

Serving Suggestions: Let cool for 20 minutes before serving.

Preparation & Cooking Tips: Use superfine almond flour.

Chocolate Pudding Cake

Preparation Time: 5 minutes
Cooking Time: 30 minutes
Servings: 6

Ingredients:

- 2 cups water

Chocolate cake

- 1/3 cup coconut flour
- 2/3 cup almond flour
- 1/3 cup cocoa powder
- 2 tablespoons keto sweetener
- 1 teaspoon baking powder
- 1 cup butter
- 3 eggs, beaten
- 1 teaspoon vanilla extract
- 1 cup coconut milk

Chocolate sauce

- 1 tablespoon keto sweetener
- 5 tablespoons cocoa powder
- 1 cup boiling water

Method:

1. In a bowl, mix the flours, cocoa powder, sweetener and baking powder.
2. Stir in the butter, eggs, vanilla extract and coconut milk.
3. Mix well.
4. Pour mixture into a baking pan.
5. Mix the chocolate sauce ingredients in another bowl.
6. Spread this on top of the mixture.
7. Cover pan with foil.
8. Add water to the Ninja Foodi.
9. Place steamer inside the pot.
10. Put the baking pan on top of the steamer.

11. Secure the lid.
12. Cook on high for 30 minutes.
13. Release pressure quickly.

Serving Suggestions: Top with whipped cream.

Preparation & Cooking Tips: Use unsweetened cocoa powder.

Conclusion

In a nutshell, ketosis is our body's survival mode when it can't get its usual sugar fuel.

By starving the body of carbs, we force it to undergo the metabolic state of ketosis. The keto diet is tailored to keep the body in the state of ketosis to take advantage of its many health benefits.

The ketogenic diet can help many people, especially those with Type 2 diabetes, which affects around 400 million worldwide.

The rise of diabetes and obesity, especially in younger people, has become a global issue. This highlights the importance of our diet in our overall health and wellness.

The keto diet has shown to be highly effective for weight loss. When done right, it has the potential to improve brain functions and neurological disorders.

At the end of the day, it is a highly restrictive diet and may not be for everyone.

It is essential that we consult a health professional before we make drastic changes to our diets.

Once you get a go signal from your doctor, the keto diet can definitely make positive changes in your health and overall life.

CPSIA information can be obtained
at www.ICGtesting.com
Printed in the USA
BVHW010630040121
596926BV00007B/161